MINDSOLASTA

think. change. illuminate.

# PRAISE FOR MINDSOLASTA

"Mindsolasta- Well articulated book in layman terms which many of the authors in the recent times fail at. I am pleased at the simplicity of the book its language and non-repetitive lines. It's an amazing work, All the articles are crisp shot and simple. Personally, I enjoyed reading it and definitely would suggest everyone. Mr. Paul Raj and Ms. Aishwarya Sibey has channelled brilliantly.. my best wishes for your success..!"

—**Nagabhushan. A,** Principal SCVVHS, Co-founder and secretary 'Wings Education Trust'

"The book focusses on mental framework which all of us go through once in our lifetime. Aptly structured and presented. Amazing writing."

—**Dr. Saumya,** MDS in Prosthodontics

"I thoroughly enjoyed reading Mindsolasta. There's a lot to learn from this book. It really had a good impact on me. I felt positive when I finished reading it. The inclusion of those amazing quotes is indeed great! The articles covered in this book are exemplary. Overall, this is a book, which helps us to work on ourselves and build self-love. I'm genuinely grateful to you for bringing up such a good content."

—**Shabana,** Student at Jyoti Nivas College Autonomous

"A must read for all, the book spreads hope, gives practical tools to bring positive changes, very insightful and gripping whilst changing perspectives! A good read!"

—**Esha Sanghvi,** M.Sc. Psychology Student, Indian Institute of Psychology and Research

"Mindsolasta explores how powerful the positive thinking can bring up a transformation in your life in unpleasant situations. Reading this book wakes up your inner strength which helps you to stay positive and spread happiness to the people surrounding you. Each quote and article will take you to the different steps you can follow as stressful situations bring your life down. It gives an idea of how important is the children's mental health especially during the pandemic and also how the counselling could impact your life ahead. Mindsolasta inn depth make you understand the significance of mental health to have a meaningful life and changes what you think impossible to practically possible things through the presence of mind and hope."

—**Dr. Smruthi. S,** BDS

"The title of the book is catchy and attractive, and the topics of the book are well thought off. The content is easy to comprehend for most age groups and keeps the reader curiously glued to know more. Positive psychology is the need of the hour due to the rise in Mental health issues during the unprecedented COVID 19 which reflects in your writing and equal justice has been done to all the topics. Problematic Gender Role Stereotyping interested me a lot as the facts divulged in the writing was not known to me and took me by surprise , specially the fact that crying is a stress buster. Here's wishing you all the best for your first book and blessings for more. As the saying goes 'Pen is mightier than Sword' so continue to pen your expression. Love & Luck."

—**Dr. Sagareeka Roy Bhatia,** Educational Thought Leader & International Ambassador for Human Rights & World Peace

"Mindsolasta is such an important read during these times. Covid-19 came in like a tsunami and caused a lot of destruction for which we cannot do anything. Quarantine has made some people positive and some of us vulnerable and this book talk about how not to get vulnerable through positive psychology which mainly concentrates on individuals and societal well-being. A must-read for each and every one as it talks about various issues and how to cope with them, which is very important."

—**Laasya Priya,** Student at Christ University, Bangalore

"Dear Aishwarya Sibey and Paul Raj,

You have incurred a lot of hard work in it, it's really an amazing episode. Along with hundreds of quotes and reflections of in and out of human psychological dynamics: The mindfulness, positive attitude, counselling, the relationship between stress and sleep, the healing power of dancing etc are imbibed and compiled very effectively as well as efficiently. In total, it is an eye opener to the stressed minds. It's a beautiful work with research bent of mind which inspires the young minds revealing expression of a human personality. Hearty congratulations and regards to you. We whole heartedly wish you for your future endeavours."

—**V Manjula,** President and Founder, Trustee Institute of Brain and Behaviour Research Foundation (R) Bangalore

"Mindsolasta reflects the passion and efforts of young advocates of mental health. The book makes an easy read, and I hope it truly helps create a sensitised awareness, making the readers 'think, change and illuminate' attitudes towards mental health. The initiative of writing such a book is truly commendable and serves as a reminder for us to work towards making mental health a priority for all!"

—**Roshni Sondhi,** Psychologist, Fortis Healthcare

"Mindsolasta by Paul Raj and Aishwarya Sibey is a wonderful resource speaking on mental health especially in the challenging times of COVID-19 pandemic. The book gives a peek into the basic tenets of positive psychology and counselling. This book can be used as a reference for introduction towards the general concepts of psychology for the larger population and a self-help guide to maintain holistic wellbeing. The strength of the book lies in a clear, precise, non-technical style of writing focussing on the most basic aspects of mental health."

—**Dr. Venkatesh Babu GM,** Consultant Psychiatrist, Fortis Hospital Bangalore & **Ms. Akanksha Pandey,** Consultant Clinical Psychologist, Fortis Healthcare Bangalore

# MINDSOLASTA

think. change. illuminate.

*Paul Raj & Aishwarya Sibey*

Inkfeathers Publishing

Mindsolasta- think. change. illuminate.
Paul Raj & Aishwarya Sibey
Print Edition

First Published & Printed in India in 2021
Inkfeathers Publishing
New Delhi 110095


ISBN 978-81-950205-0-8



www.inkfeathers.com

*A special thanks to Dad, Mom, Rithika Vinod and Konaukanjoli Chakravathy*

# CONTENTS



## Articles

# PREFACE

*"Positive Psychology aims to catalyze a change in psychology from a preoccupation only with repairing the worst things in life to also building the best qualities in life."*

*-Martin Seligman*

Amidst the coronavirus induced lockdown, I did not know what to do, and with a blank mind and dreary eyes stared at the empty roads from the balcony of my house, with silence and fear accompanying my thoughts of what is next? I wondered; will our future dreams come true or are they going to be shattered into many pieces all because of this pandemic?

Then, there came the thought of why not take this pandemic to take as a challenge and create more opportunities by spreading some positivity into the soul of every individual and bring the butterflies out of each one of us, in these bland times of the pandemic. There came a purpose to do something for the people around the world.

Mindsolasta is written from my passion with the intent of spreading some positivity in society. It is also about raising awareness on how important 'Positive Psychology' is for an individual in today's catastrophe-struck world. The primary aim is to surpass the negativity, cherish the positivity, and encourage all of us to introspect and retrospect simultaneously.

Positive Psychology is a relatively new field discipline but has spread rapidly in the last year as everyone has grappled with their demons during this time. In a time of despair, we have all tried to hang onto the shreds of normalcy, and my mission is to use Positive Psychology help all of us cope with this "new normal" as everyone calls it.

While it has not been an easy year, and it certainly will not get easier as fast as we are hoping for it to, it is my opinion that by practising this discipline we can learn to overlook the negatives and instead focus on the positives. If we learn to develop our strengths, we can gradually come to terms with if not overcome our weaknesses and live a life of better quality and more meaning.

Positive Psychology has been claimed to be ignorant for focusing on only the good instead of the bad, but it is in fact a process which rights all wrongs too. It just chooses to use the prettier path to recovery instead of taking the rough path.

By encouraging those who are moderately or barely hurt to work on themselves, Positive Psychology tries to improve everyone's morale and is about practising mindfulness, gratitude, and general happiness. By doing this, we can all be better versions of ourselves and coexist with fewer clashes and conflicts.

The focus of Positive Psychology in a simple summary is:

1. Positive Experiences of happiness, inspiration, and such positive feelings.

2. Positive States and Traits like compassion, resilience, and such practices.

3. Positive Community and Institutions – you spread your positive state among the people you work with or live with.

These three focuses are divided into three levels, the Subjective level, the Individual level, and the Group level. These three levels are the way to ensuring that positive psychology spreads among many people and can impact many lives at once. By practising it by ourselves and in a community, we also help many people out of their state of despair.

Psychology as a field historically shed light and spend time researching only for those who suffer, the average people became weaker and this is when it was realised that normal people should also learn how to make the best of their lives. That is where Positive Psychology comes in. It aims to counter the belief that psychology is only for the mentally ill. It gives attention to the average person so they too can live in a better state.

There are many ways to practice this discipline. You can start by writing a gratitude journal or expressing your joy for the smaller things to those around you. As time passes, you will find this gratitude which may have felt like a task in the beginning gradually becoming a habit which comes without any hesitation.

If you simply compliment people or tell them how you enjoy having them around, you also start a chain of what I like to call "Good Actions". This chain helps bring smiles to many faces and lead to a domino effect due to which many people can be better versions of who they were previously.

It is when you start to understand what makes life worth living that you truly can push yourself to boundaries you never thought you would break past. And it is only when you push yourself that you really start living.

Positive Psychology also brings benefits to many aspects of one's life. It helps in social wellbeing, allows you to get comfortable with how you are feeling and offers a space to you to vent your darker thoughts. As you expel these negative thoughts, you begin to create the room needed to harbour positive feelings and thoughts and in turn become a better human being.

Another benefit of practising Positive Psychology is it teaches you to appreciate the present with more fervour. Instead of looking onto the future, you begin to see the value of the moment you are in and savour the now more than the possibilities of an unpromised tomorrow. As this happens you will also become a pleasure to be around as your positive outlook on all matters will reach to the people around you.

Meditation, breathing exercises and hot tea will all guide you on this path as you try to get in sync with your innermost thoughts and regulate the energy you give out. Mindsolasta will also see you through this transformation from good to better to best. And as you improve, so will your surroundings and the people around you. This journey may not be the shortest, but it is worth the resulting joy you will receive. And it is one filled with sights worth admiring and being thankful for.

I can only hope, that as time passes you begin to practice these rituals more often and learn to indulge yourself in smaller joys like taking a walk on a breezy day or having a cup of a warm beverage as it rains outside. I also hope that you and your loved one's practice mindfulness together to overcome the blockade of dreariness which may be weighing you down at this very moment.

I wish that you will be able to dance in the rain or indoors to the beats of your favourite songs and be grateful for every breath you can take and every sight you can take in with your eyes. As you grow, may you see how beautiful the world and its people are even with all its challenges and flaws.

And finally, I pray that each one of you can undergo a metamorphosis to become your best and most beautiful selves. This future version of yours, be proud of it but do not forget to appreciate who you are today too.

Hope you have a great time through the journey of this book.

Signing off,

Paul Raj

# “Quotes”

“

Transform your differences into your greater strengths.

The present circumstance is determined on your journey, not your destination.

Self- care is the power you give to nourish your own self.

A little girl with vision today is to be empowered woman tomorrow.

In between the social sea of life, it takes courage to fight for the freedom of the mind.

Thinking is the soul of the mind.

”

“

Every little change counts.

Illuminate the igniting mind.

Though our branches grow in different directions, our roots remain as one. Each of us remain priceless!

Your identity solely rests on the reflection of the world that you're a daughter.

Being pessimistic is a choice. But being optimistic is also a choice that gives more energy to thrive in our lives. Be optimistic, be energised, always thrive.

”

"

A single pinch of hope is still a powerful place to be in.

Literacy is our shade for hope and well-being.

A great teacher is always, a true mentor of our hearts, and a quintessence of juxtaposition.

Connect with yourself to connect with others.

You are the sailor of your life, and therefore you decide your destination.

In the depths of despair, mental health requires more of unashamed confer, to find one's strength within.

"

“

A single smile can affect overall mental health.

A proud Indian with freedom of mind.

It’s ok to have a fall when it leads to empowering learning.

When the sun goes down, the moon comes up. Don’t lose hope!

A few relations on earth never die.

A mental health first aid helps in battling an array of negativity.

”

"

Take a mental break and create your own happy hours.

It's ok if you take pills for your mental well-being. End pill shaming!

Experience is what you bring up, not what is given to you.

Unmute suppression. Speak up!

A therapist is who knows all about you, yet still stands to support & help you.

Talking out today for a brighter tomorrow. The power of counselling!

"

“

Thankfulness is a form of authentic happiness.

Practice nourishing self-love!

Healing occurs while you integrate from trauma.

Don’t make the anxiety yours, face the crowd with confidence!

Assessment begins with a referral!

Think what went wrong, change the situation, and illuminate your thoughts.

”

“

Never fear in what you want to accomplish.

Believe you will heal.

Develop the skill of appreciating every smallest thing.

Do not dig yourself deep into the burrows of depression.
Seek Help!

If it's a disorder, it's not the end of everything. Do not be ashamed of it, instead talk it out!

Eradicate self-hate and build a ravishing strength.

”

"

Learn the art of appreciating yourself.

Do not judge based on your mental illness. Fight it out!

Speak up, before up attempt to give up.

Grow stronger, beyond your illness.

Love and support all people, regardless of orientation.

It isn't about what's wrong with you, but what went wrong with you.

Life is ironic, choose to stay kind.

"

“

Freedom comes from bringing yourself!

It’s absolutely ok if you’re not perfect, just stay yourself!

The best apology is to forgive and not to repeat the mistake.

Stay genial with yourself.

The moon is the best example, that even in the darkest it stands bright.

Develop fortitude.

”

"

Shoot away your ego with gratitude!

Be a flawsome in your frame of life.

Create your own masterpiece.

Be your own juxtaposition.

Be your own painter of your everyday life.

Please yourself, not anyone else.

Illuminate your thoughts.

"

"

Habituate to mindfulness.

It doesn't matter how you are now but matters what you will be next.

Choose your self-talk wisely.

You're rich when you receive self-satisfaction.

Bring out the spark in you.

Own your degree of self-love.

Invest in happiness.

"

“

It’s ok for men to breakdown or feel for.

Share some love to the entities of mother earth.

There will be a rainbow after every rainy day!

Failure is the door to success!!

There will be stars after a rainy night!

Pour your own sunshine.

Be stronger than your fear.

”

"

Dance while everybody else walks.

Create your own sparkle on the way and a leave a lasting light.

Inner beauty and confidence do not require to make up.

It's ok to say NO. The power of assertiveness!

Be the unicorn between the horses.

Let's talk about mental health and empower it.

In the expense of quarantine, create your own bliss.

"

“

Dream it, live it!

If you can’t explore out, explore in you.

Believe in what you can.

There is no shame in dealing with schizophrenia or mental disorder.

Mental health is as important as any other illness.

Give yourself a credit in the journey of mental wellbeing.

Nourish your thoughts and feelings, it's important.

”

"

Feelings are sometimes the communication of the soul. Pay attention to it!

It might be a small thing to help an animal, but it's a big thing for them.

You don't have to be fully drowned to seek help; a small sign is enough to seek immediate help which will lead to prevention of severity!

Once you set a destination in google maps, it changes the route depending on the roadblocks. It doesn't change the destination. So, in life, be flexible enough to change the route but not the destination.

"

“

Be your own beautiful.

Penchant your own self.

From dark clouds, we get precious water, from dark mines we get valuable jewels, and from our darkest trials comes our best.

Life is like a Rubix cube, it's in our hands to fix it. Reach to your therapist!

You may be a bud today, but tomorrow you will bloom. Be patient!

”

"

Accept criticism and appreciation. They help you heal.

Positive thinking is not only about expecting the best to happen, but it's also about accepting, whatever happens, is for the best.

Life is sometimes like the keys of the piano, there must be bright and dark keys to get the harmony for the tune.

It's ok to take your time and heal. Be patient!

Mental illness is nothing to be ashamed of, neither is talking about it.

"

Do not dread on your illness, take timely help from your therapist.

End the stigma of mental illness!

Don't travel with others criticism on you, instead make it a journey to learn from them. Keep going!

It's absolutely alright to relax from a day, a mental break is necessary!

If you fail, it's not the end. It's just you have found ways to work out.

"

The handle to the door of the heart is from inside and not from out. You have the key.

Mental illness is not a failure.

Heaven and Hell are not geographical locations, instead, they are our own very own thoughts, actions and behaviours that create heaven or hell for us.

Fight for your battle every day. Do not quit!

Therapy defines something that you can work with.

The secret of life is to get started and not to stop trying.

"

“

You might be going through mental illness, but you’re not your mental illness. All you need is an unashamed conversation.

You’re the warrior in the battle called life. Face it with all strength!

Choose to take each day with love.

Life is balanced with two magical poles, positive and negative, you got to choose which dominates the most in your life.

It’s ok to have a breakdown, just don’t stay down there with broken pieces. Let it out and refocus on your goals.

”

“

Your negative thinking is not your personality. Let it go!

If you’re looking for someone, know that you are enough.

Call yourself a warrior, fight for your mental health!

Seeking help is a courageous step, and taking that wise step is a powerful one.

Every day begins with an act of courage: accepting yourself.

Keep going ahead, as always, knowing that you are worthy of a happy life.

”

“

Thinking begins with your ownership of choosing the right thoughts.

The most wonderful people are those who keep trying and believe they can do it.

If you want to swim, you got to cross the tides.

Reminder: Just because you had a bad day, doesn’t mean it’s the same tomorrow.

Your positive mental health is essential.

Sometimes positive mental health leads to self-care.

”

"

Crying isn't a sign of weakness unless you keep moving on after every cry.

Positivity may not make the world happy, but it makes the ride worthwhile.

Get independence from the need for perfection.

Breathe to live for yourself.

Try loving yourself and see the magic.

In the journey of life, the answers for your struggle is given as you move on.

"

“

Even from a thunder, songs of hope can be called.

You might be afraid of your own mind but give it some charm with hope.

It’s all about your view which should be important to you.

Never let your emotions overpower productivity.

The elevator to happiness is your choice of thoughts.

Inner peace begins when you do not let your emotions control you.

”

"

Let the incredible colours out of you.

Understanding your own feelings is art.

No one can make you feel less worthy.

Your cognition begins with what you allow.

Love yourself, beyond hope, faith, rules, and fear.

Remind yourself that you are precious.

Empathy defines your strength.

"

"

Do not be sad if you fail, it's just a steppingstone to bring more colour out of you.

Celebrate the child in you.

Only with the crack, the sprout grows to be a plant.

Learning and listening from others should be a great practice.

Unplug yourself from fear.

Don't let your fear be your identity.

"

"

The journey within is the most precious one. Think positive!

The art of extreme care is self-care.

If you possess the ability to be kind, make yourself the priority.

Make the integrity of your path.

Grow where you were sown.

Make your scars to be your strength.

"

"

Exaggerate your power to overcome the storms.

Thinking happy leads to a path of feeling happy.

Enjoy every moment as it will never be back. Find happiness everywhere!

Thinking makes everything different. Think positive!

You get to decide if you get discouraged from your downs or learn from those.

Do not be stuck somewhere you don't belong. Be the change!

"

“

Alter your living by altering your thoughts.

Positive thinking is itself a good exercise.

Time has a wonderful way of explaining the meaning of living.

Reflect your courage, not your fears.

Fix your thinking, the problems will move its own pace.

Taking steps in life is important, even though the steps taken are shaky.

”

"

Self- care is how you love yourself.

Keep looking for the colours when your life turns dark.

Therapy is because you deserve it.

Explore solutions that overcome your anxiety.

Recognise the signs of your behaviour.

Play positive with your problem-solving skills.

Analyse when you start catastrophising

"

"

Practice colouring your mindfulness.

Brainstorm solutions to overcome the challenges.

Process praise on yourself.

It's all in your mind, train to think positively.

Practice small acts of kindness.

You control how you want to treat yourself.

Overcome everything that overcomes you.

"

"

Appreciate yourself for how resilience you have been all this while.

Look how much you've already managed to adapt to.

It's ok if you miss your old self.

Give yourself permission to step back from everything that caused anxiety.

Normalize that you can surf through the tides.

Paint your mental health with your beautiful mind and soul.

"

"

Do not give discounts on your self-care.

Start grounding at the moment.

Your mind is a warrior. Keep fighting!

It's the mind that speaks.

Communicate your need clearly.

It's ok to say no to what puts you down.

Helps your mind to see your self-worth.

"

"

Try to encourage yourself and see what happens.

A little consideration to your inner self will do the work of moving on.

Healing is a magical process, it takes strength, it takes love, it takes practice.

The ride may seem like a ride on the hill but remember once you reach the destination it's a beautiful view. Don't quit!

A calm mind is a beautiful state of happiness.

"

“

Adhere to think positively.

Don’t cage yourself with negative emotions.

Your mental health matters. Listen to your mind’s chatter.

Eat healthily and think healthy.

Therapy helps in relating better with yourself and others.

Be like a candle, even if it’s broken into two its lights.

Embrace your weakness into your strengths.

”

"

To start something new you need to adapt to change.

Once a bipolar doesn't mean you are forever. Illuminate your thoughts!

If you are a caterpillar today, remember you will be a butterfly tomorrow. Be patient!

You can't stop the tides, but you can learn to swim through them.

Your mind and body will treat you the way you let it. Inspire yourself.

"

"

Unknot your fears one by one.

Filter your thoughts to see good in every circumstance

Along the way build some strength to overcome the catastrophe.

Someone who likes you will lift you in every situation. Be the one to your own self. Be you!

Self-love is a beautiful form of love.

Being expressive is a great gift.

"

“

Bring yourself together because you are your own sunshine.

Being different doesn’t mean your worthless, it means your incredibly unique.

All you need is patience, wait for the wonderful outcome.

Every individual on this universe have their own responsibilities, but the first responsibility should be always to take care of your mental health.

Putting yourself in another state is a mindset.

”

"

Where there is positive thinking there is a positive attitude.

Sympathy and empathy are forms of healthy thinking.

Flourish your positive vibes.

Your thinking reflects your appealing personality style.

Mental health can be survived only with positive healing.

Remember you came this far, so you can go even far.

Find the light when everything fades. Stay hopeful!

"

"

Never start degrading yourself because of your bad day.

Nothing should stop you from putting yourself first.

Spread the good vibes in you.

Move ahead your life is promising to be flamboyant.

If you are taking medications, remember still you are no less to anyone. Believe in yourself!

It shouldn't cost you to be kind. Stay kind to all!

Understand that being different means being unique. Everyone is unique!

"

"

Do anything that makes your inner self smile.

Your feelings are essential; give them some love and care.

You can attend therapy even when you want to have a better understanding of yourself and others.

Hear the voice in you and communicate wisely.

Let your worth not fluctuate.

Make self-love eternal. Love yourself!

Your more important than anyone's judgement on you.

"

"

Don't store your feelings like in a closed container. Express!

You don't have to wait to start something that makes you feel warm.

During the days of insecurity remind yourself that you can beat the storm.

If there is no crack, there is no growth. The power of healing!!

It doesn't matter if you are happy only with the help of anti-depressants.

"

“

Embrace good things with both arms.

Pay close attention to what makes you happy.

The world needs you to pour your gratitude out.

Therapy is not just sharing.

Sometimes breaking into parts can be a great beginning.

Love yourself even when someone says NO.

Remember that you are strong, you have the capacity to thrive.

”

“

A psychiatrist is not only the one who helps in understanding others but importantly your own self.

When you fall apart, recentre yourself.

Do not apologise for your imperfections.

Build an extravagant friendship with your soul and mind.

When melancholy hits you, explore your creativity and watch the skills spilling out.

Do not make your fear an addiction. Surf through the storm!

”

"

The power of accepting yourself is to love yourself unconditionally.

Patience is a form of therapy. Practice it!

Your failure is your strength for the betterment.

Be mindful of the present, the rest will fall in its place.

You don't have to apologise for your mental illness.

Make yourself the most valuable.

Send love to all those struggling in despair.

"

“

Find reasons for your living.

Vent out, do not get obsessed with your anxiety.

It’s ok if all you did was calming down your irrational thoughts.

If you believe in yourself and strive for the best, you will lead an optimistic life.

Don’t let your past overflow you.

Do not take a ride with wrong things, just learn from them, and keep going.

”

Adapt to practice gratitude every day. Remember to do it even when you fall apart.

Just don't dream for what you want, thrive for it.

Let your attitude of seeing things determine your ability.

It's absolutely ok if you relapse but never quit.

Show off that you matter first.

Nobody can lift you to other than yourself. Believe in you!!

“

Keep trying and you will keep moving at your own pace.

Don’t make the consequence easier, you must become tough.

Make your aim to work out the impossible.

Always be prepared to create a road to recovery.

Spread plenty of goodness wherever you go.

Be tough, let the storm not overcome you.

”

"

Being able to learn the pain is the attribute of the strong.

The seasons shall pass, so shall the hard days.

Forgiving will define your goodness, even if the victim regrets his mistake or not.

Surround yourself with all the good entities of the earth.

Try, try, keep trying, for success will find its way. The potential for success!

"

# Articles

# 1

# A CLOSER HOME, A NATIONWIDE LOCKDOWN: PRECIOUS DAYS SPENT WITHIN THE THATCHED WALLS

"Potatoes stored for the winter in a dark cellar would produce small, thin shoots that grew to the distant light of a faraway window."

~ *Carl Rogers*

Man, an optimistic animal, however bad his environmental conditions are, he will still strive to grow and develop, just like the potato shoots in a dark cellar. Staying between the four thatched walls during this quarantine is like a ride on the edge of the knife for every individual and family as this environmental catastrophe has instigated a huge social, financial, political, religious, and psychological imbalance. The disruption of normalcy in school and college life, denuded jobs and salary cuts, the anxiety created in the world grappled with this insidious virus, and the psychological scars of social distancing can be just as gruesome. Quarantine like this can result in

PTSD symptoms like irritability, anxiety, loss of interest, depression, and insomnia, the effects of which can be enduring.

These uncertainties call for one and all 'Think, Change and Illuminate'. We must be mindful of each other and show the highest self-esteem to enhance self-care and family-care. We need to understand that this devastating process of change can be an ordeal for all but at the same time, a positive approach can lead one and all to a beautiful and happy destination. To direct the winds is out of our control, but by adjusting the sails and working from home, introspection ("looking within") at this juncture should be held high. "He who knows others is wise; he who knows himself is enlightened" (Lao Tzu). Every positive sprout needs to be recognized and valued through our doors of life.

To weaken or detect the onset of any mental health implications, we open our minds to something as simple and generous as the beauty and melody in nature -the birds' chirping in harmony, the sound of the ocean, and the silence nature has to offer. A special mention has to be made to all the front-line workers, our real heroes of this pandemic - doctors, nurses, cops, and others who, disregarding their mental health state, are on duty so that we citizens can relax at home.

I have been spending my days of quarantine with research, learning new academic writing skills, and enhancing the quality of knowledge. Additionally, keeping a track of at least five To-Do-List, reading, writing a gratitude journal, and cooking with love, being faithful to work, connecting socially with friends and relatives, finding ways to rekindle the inner child in me, and spending some quality time for myself are some of the ways I opted to hit the pandemic stress and create positive vibes. Such habits can help us inculcate new psychological strengths such as resilience which can further guide one through a blooming path towards a positive quarantine.

It is very normal to feel detached from oneself when confined to your own thoughts for a number of days. And that is why it is all the more important to keep a check on one's mental health and try to move on with thinking positively.

Any warning signs, if observed, it is always good to reach out for help. "Prevention is Better than Cure", always.

# 2

# STAYING HOME AND STAYING POSITIVE: A UNIVERSAL COMPASSION THROUGH HUMANNESS

"Only if we understand, can we care.
Only if we care, will we help.
Only if we help, shall they be saved."
~ *Jane Goodall*

At this quarantine time, my own thoughts overwhelm me and guide me to explore my inner self. I obliged by allotting my time and energy constructively like learning a new skill, engaging in new activities, sketching, dancing, flowing to the tune of the music, doing research, writing poems and blogs, and also doing an online course that could help me in improving learning skills and replenish my knowledge.

During these anxious and uncertain days, varied psychological disturbances such as anxiety, helplessness, irritability, stress, and negative thinking have interrupted my peace of mind and harmony many a times. But whenever these signs of melancholy engulf me, there happens other events that have led me to see humanity from a different perspective. I am astonished to witness humanity through my caring family, friendly neighbourhood, and ever-reliable friends as they share their love even from distant pathways with utmost genuineness and that creates memories to last forever.

In retrospect, there are so many unique memories that make me realise how important these days are for us as we finally understand the worth of others and their love that has protected me these days. It is now that I understand that this challenging face of social distancing has made me realise how important each decision of others is in my life. This is the time when we cannot only make ourselves happy but also share positive vibes to our surroundings and everyone in it. Such positive approaches will have a positive influence on us to grow, with peace and harmony.

It is essential that we practice mindfulness to nourish our inner selves while we are conversing with others as well as ourselves. I realised during this crisis time that love for oneself increases positive feelings and mindset. It is also important to learn the skill of open- mindedness, as this allows us to listen to others without any judgment or criticisms. It teaches us that every individual is unique and dynamic in their own way irrespective of their status, literacy, colour, creed, or speech. It is said, "life is the sum of all your choices" (Albert Camus). The way we speak and communicate defines us and it is important to hone our mind into growing beautifully by learning self-acceptance and acquiring different skills from the universe.

The kindness that we show ourselves and others will lead to success and adaptation in our lives. Such enriching kindness should not be showered towards mankind alone but also animals as well. This period of social distancing has made me value my pet and also it has helped me realise how a pet can help you beat sadness. If an individual can mingle with an animal with love and care, I consider it a reflection of true love, as William Shakespeare says, "One beautiful heart is better than a thousand beautiful faces." This is the expected process of giving back to the universe, what we have received in kindness. It is one of the most wonderful experiences that we may not realize when they are with us but in our painful journey, they make us feel their presence. I wish that every human being share their love and care not only towards humans but also to our ever-grateful animals and to shower them by the innate kindness and mindfulness that we have received. A part or whole of our soul remains far from awakening until we love animals. Every animal on earth has every right to be here and cared, just like you and me. As Albert Einstein has said, *"The world is a dangerous place, not because of those who do evil, but because of those who look on and do nothing."* The father of our nation, Mahatma Gandhi has beautifully put it: *"The greatness of a nation can be judged by the way its animals are treated."* Let's not forget that a hundred years from now, it will not matter the sort of house we lived in, the money we had, the technology we developed, the positions we held, the type of cars we drove, but the world may be a different place because we were important in the lives of animals. For, universal kindness, like a boomerang, always return.

# 3

# WHY TO BE MINDFUL?

"The best way to capture moments is to pay attention. This is how we cultivate mindfulness."

~ *Jon Kaba- Zinn*

To be mindful is to be present at the moment without any judgements, to pay complete attention to mind, body and the environment surrounding us. Life can be full of ups and downs; our mind can be distorted with lots of thoughts which may impact both positively and negatively.

Mindfulness benefits psychologically, cognitively, and physically as well, it helps in rewiring the circumstances. Mindfulness reduces stress levels and anxiety disorders, increases the level of happiness, improves memory and creativity, and develops the immune system. Indeed, mindfulness also increases the capacity of human brain functioning and cognitive processes, helps in better understanding of managing emotions and feelings. All of these factors lead to adapting and flourishing of a healthy well-being.

Practising meditation succour in reducing depression, anxiety, trauma, and results in improved concentration and communication.

We can learn to be mindful anywhere and anytime by observing and focusing internally and externally.

At the workplace, schools and other institutions, mindfulness favours in boasting rational thinking ability and encourages in focusing on the task. Mindfulness technique is now in a heightened state with people adapting it for an improved lifestyle. Practising mindfulness gives a promising result. As Mother Theresa says, "Be happy at the moment, that's enough. Each moment is all we need, not more."

How to practice mindfulness?

- By focusing on the present and avoiding and worrying about the past or future situations.
- Paying attention to what is happening in and around us, keenly focusing on our feelings, thoughts, sounds, etc.
- Practicing mediating techniques, listening to music, gardening, cooking, and other mindful methods help to keep the mind and body calm and at its own pace.

Learning to incorporate mindfulness may not happen in a day or so, it takes time and practice. It is equally important to adapt to practising a mindfulness technique to build a healthy lifestyle and mental healing. Cultivating mindfulness is one of the most powerful forms of therapy in today's world.

# 4

# THE RELATIONSHIP BETWEEN STRESS AND SLEEP

"Tired mind don't plan well. Sleep first, plan later."

~ *Walter Reisch*

Many of the stressors impact our sleep patterns in today's modern life. Poor sleep patterns can lead to having a bad/negative mood, low/no energy level, lack of concentration or poor eating habits. Sleep deprivation or chronic sleeping patterns increases risk in depression, strokes, obesity, heart, and kidney diseases and leads to a heightened state of arousal. Stress levels and lack of sleep leads to both physical and mental damage, sleep and stress are double trouble. Sleep-related disorders are majorly caused due to stress and anxiety issues. Though, maybe a certain amount of stress can help in motivating to improve work performance, chronic stress can disrupt an entire day's performance.

Sleep acts as a stress reliever, but stress induces sleep disturbances which can lead to sleep disorders like Insomnia, obstructive sleep apnea, narcolepsy, sleepwalking, etc. As Danzae Pace says, "Stress is the trash of modern life- we all generate it but if you don't dispose it of properly, it will pile up and overtake your life."

Chronic stress is something like being in a perpetual state of danger, which leads to increased stress and anxiety. Stress can adversely affect sleep quality and the duration to fall asleep. Certain hormonal changes and imbalances, medications, caffeine, alcohol, and other drugs can also impact sleep patterns.

- Techniques to reduce stress and sleep better:
- Developing an assertive behaviour
- Developing healthy eating habits and well-balanced food
- Exercise
- Practising mindfulness techniques
- Reducing caffeine intake
- Avoid procrastination
- Adapt to breathing techniques
- Spend time with family and friends

Practicing these techniques might help in reducing stress and in sleeping better, yet sometimes, if the stress exceeds to an uncontrollable level, then taking a precautionary from the doctor is always advisable.

# 5

# THE POWER OF COUNSELLING

"The only person who is educated is the one who has learned how to learn to change."

~ *Carl Roger*

What comes to mind when we tell counselling?

Counselling is a very powerful tool and an incredible skill to acquire. It helps in navigating away the negative things in life by starting to adapt to positivity in every situation. From the ancestral times there had been something called 'giving guidance' which is now developed into 'counselling' through the professionals.

There is nothing wrong in seeking for help, all of us require some help at some point in life. Counselling helps in examining emotions and psychological problems. Counselling ensures support, provides resources and information to deal with any kind of situation that life throws at us. It is all about sharing and engaging in a conversation without passing any judgement or but by being neutral. As all that is shared is completely confidential. Therefore, it helps in talking out openly about anything, in case if the counsellor understands that the client's life is in danger, then the counsellor may have to reveal certain information to the person who is trustworthy and close to the client, because safety is always the first priority.

Henceforth, counselling enables the individual to manage the passages of life, to develop coping strategies, to see the issues more objectively by coming in terms with the past experiences and helps in building self-esteem and confidence so as to think and deal assertively. As Eleanor Roosevelt says, "You gain strength, courage, and confidence by every experience in which you really stop to look at fear in the face." You are able to say to yourself, 'I lived through this horror. I can take the next thing that comes along.'

All that we need to do is ask for help and understand that there is no shame in asking for help or to seek a friendly ear. Asking or seeking for help is a one of the courageous steps you will be taking, the time is all yours in talking what is important to you by offering safe space.

Nobody in this world is alone, together we can make ample amounts of difference, resulting in a happier and better life.

# 6

# THE IMPORTANCE OF UNDERSTANDING EMOTIONS

"Emotions are the keys to learning, the keys to imprinting. The stronger the emotion, the more clearly the experience is learned."

~ *Clotaire Rapallie*

It is important to learn and understand how emotions and feelings manifest and shape us. Emotions not only help us connect with others; it also helps in connecting with oneself. Every living being is gifted with emotions and feelings. Feeling is something which is regarded as the primary aspect of life. Emotions play a key role in how we think and behave. Different elements of emotion play different roles in our life such as love, joy, sadness, anger, disgust, etc. Experiencing these varied emotions can lead to motivation or anxiety. In some of the circumstances, we might experience positive emotions and minimize the negative emotions. For example: Meeting a friend might give a positive feeling and help us overcome all the negativity we experienced that day. Naturalist Darwin believed that emotions are adaptations which allows both humans and animals to survive to reproduce.

The purpose of our emotions:

Emotions help us to thrive, to make decisions, survive and allow others to understand us and us to understand them. They are a powerful tool that helps us interact meaningfully in our social sea of life. Emotions produce different kinds of physiological, biological, and cognitive changes.

There are 3 paths to an emotion:

1. A subjective component which is how we experience the emotion.
2. A physiological component which is how our bodies react to the emotion.
3. An expressive component which is how we behave in the report to the emotion.

Managing both positive and negative emotions is essential for having a healthy lifestyle. Independence is grounded in expressing emotions by acknowledging and experiencing them. Expressing emotions and reacting to them is good for our mental and physical health. Emotions are the universal language to understand people and relate to them better by making the relationship more meaningful.

# 7

# THE POWER OF THANKFULNESS AND GRATITUDE

"Acknowledging the good that you already have in life is the foundation for all abundance."

~ *Eckhart Tolle*

Gratitude and thankfulness are associated with greater happiness. It is the most powerful tool that can be practised every day, by being grateful for the things you have. Thankfulness and gratitude are something that money cannot buy. We need to adapt to a mentality to chase our dreams and be grateful for it. One of the greatest success would be that we should be insanely thankful from what we have come through, the way of getting rich is through the genuine expression of these two powerful elements.

Thankfulness and gratitude are both a law of attraction and helps in relating and creating a healthier and stronger bond, there are interpersonal and intrapersonal benefits which create a correlation between mental and physical well-being. The more of positivity and good things we give, the more we receive. It keeps us in close harmony with oneself and others. Practising these two mindful elements can increase in illuminating happiness by diminishing depression and increasing resilience and pro-social behaviour which is further linked to positive attitude. As Henri Frederic Amiel says, "Thankfulness is the beginning of gratitude. Gratitude is the completion of thankfulness. Thankfulness can consist merely of words. Gratitude is shown in acts."

Mindfulness kick starts the brain and body with increased production of dopamine and serotonin. These two elements appears to be self-perpetuating and act as an anti-depressant by creating happiness and contentment by deflecting the negative attitude. Thankfulness and gratitude help in magnifying the positivity and celebrate the present. A simple 'thank you' can not only make someone's day but also lift the spirit and morale. Thankfulness and gratitude have superpowers to improve mood, make someone feel worthy, improves problem-solving skills, builds self-esteem and confidence. Grateful people are seen as the ones with a positive approach to life.

Not only words like 'thank you' and 'I'm grateful' are ways of conveying gratitude or being thankful, but an apt body language and action conveys the message in a more meaningful manner. As Mahatma Gandhi has said, "Action speaks louder than words." Let us all tune ourselves to practicing thankfulness and gratitude and seize our blessings by holding them close to our heart.

# 8

# SELF-LOVE- A STEP TOWARDS SELF-ENHANCEMENT

"It's yourself all that will stay by you, in the ride of your journey."

~ *Paul Raj*

Have you ever thought of the relationship you have with yourself? About how much love and care you shower on you like you do shower on others? Do you feel love or hatred towards yourself?

Self-love is a nourishing source that you give to yourself to grow incredibly into a uniquely beautiful being. A state of care and appreciation to oneself both psychologically and physically regardless of others love and care for you. The act of accepting oneself 'the way you are', having regards for well-being and happiness, sacrificing and being hungry for one's happiness and the healthy state of mind.

Pouring self-love and care can work like an energy booster and act as a self-motivating pill. Loving oneself doesn't mean you are selfish or the most flamboyant human being on this planet. All that it means is accepting your weakness, flaws and building some self-motivation & strength to overcome the negativity that hits you during your difficult times.

Other people's opinion on you doesn't define who you are, but it takes so much of pride and capability to be true to oneself and to have enjoyed the precious moments of who you are to you rather than who you are to others. People who are with you make an impact on your life but remember, it is you who makes the biggest impact on yourself. Your thinking and your state of well-being defines you and appreciates all the struggle that you have overcome till now. Self-love is two-fold, it is a feeling and simultaneously an action, the two of this invokes the emotion of love, and not only love but also maintains mental hygiene. It is the love you show yourself like you do show for someone else and feel good about it.

It is only by loving yourself that you can really love others. Give yourself time, have good food, read books and rest when you need it. We never know who will stay in our life and how long. All you know is you have you around for as long as you live.

Self- love should be practised throughout life, lack of self-love can increase the risk of suicide, depression, hopelessness, and low self-esteem. Lacking self-love, we not only get into a toxic relationship with ourselves but with others as well. It also affects in decision making. Therefore, every one of us needs to practice and nurture self-love. As Diane Von Furstenberg says, "It is so important to take time for yourself and find clarity. The most important relationship is the one you have with yourself."

# 9

# FOSTERING POSITIVE MENTAL HEALTH

"What mental health needs is more sunlight, more candour, more unashamed conversation."

*~ Glenn Close*

It is very important to nourish our mental health with positivity. A healthy mind and well-being can be defined as positive mental health, which encompasses feeling good about oneself, coping with daily stress, building resilience, helping the community. Mental health plays a very crucial role in every one of our life, people who possess positive mental health have some zest and enthusiasm in living their life to the fullest, they find a sense of meaning and purpose, holds a lot of self-esteem and confidence.

Having positive mental doesn't mean that we never go through any kind of downs, but it is all about how we overcome those downs and start to being resilient and move on in life. Positive mental health is all about the human mind. The psycho-social environment plays a dominant role in the individuals mental health. The standards of mental health differ from place to place, time, culture, social groups, and expectations and how the individual views the world. An individual with increased positive mental health is associated with a decreased state of depression and other mental illness and vice versa. All of us strive for our mind to be positive, buoyant, strong, and confident.

There are different ways to practice reprogramming of your mind for positive mental health:

1. Focusing on the positive- Thinking about those who have been supportive and the circumstances when you have received appreciation from others which made you happy.
2. Build problem-solving skills- It's important to know that every problem has a solution, and it's up to us on how we are going to cope and deal with them.
3. Practice gratitude-Being grateful to people, and helping others give us pleasure and make them happy too.
4. Connect with others- Creating a stronger bond with meaningful relationships, spending time with family and friends.
5. Taking a break from social media- Starting to connect physically and emotionally than virtually can make an impact on our positive mental health.
6. Exercise- Practicing some daily exercise can enhance alertness and helps in being resilient.
7. Healthy diet- It is very important to have a healthy meal and a balanced diet to stay physically and mentally fit.
8. Getting creative- Practicing art or music can help in expressing oneself and engrossing in positive energy.
9. Getting enough sleep- Getting proper rest and sleep is very essential for the mind and body and helps in detoxing the negative elements.
10. Asking for help- Seeking help from a therapist or a counsellor helps in understanding the emotions better and developing positive thinking and attitude by looking at the world optimistically.

It is important to attune our mind to positive thinking. We need to learn to live happily and to the fullest. As Mahatma Gandhi has said, "Live as if you were to die tomorrow. Learn as if you were to live forever."

# 10

# THE ART OF MINDFUL LISTENING

"The art of conversation is the art of hearing as well as being heard."

*~William Hazlitt*

Are you a mindful listener? Do you pay attention to what others are saying or are you engrossed in your own thoughts?

Mindful listening is all about paying keen attention to what others are saying without reflecting or being judgemental.

Eye contact, paraphrasing, nodding are some of the signs of mindful listening. Mindful listening is a form of meditation. Well, it is not all about being patient and being aware of things inside us and around us, whether it is inside our head, breathing or all the sounds around us, but mindful listening involves both verbal and non-verbal language.

It is important to understand that when someone shares with you it is because they are comfortable and trust you. So, it is important to always listen and understand to the individual without being cynical or shrewd. Most of the times, just talking or being with the person itself does a lot. Being there for others and listening to them without any criticisms or judgement is the most wonderful thing we can do for others.

Mindful listening needs more of dedication, contemplation. We need to show them that we are paying genuine attention and is empathetic of what is shared with us.

How to nurture it?

- Repeat and paraphrase
- Hold patience
- Be non-judgemental
- Develop to nod while listening
- Keep eye contact

Benefits of mindful listening:

- Improves physical mental
- Improves mental health
- Increases empathy
- Improves focus and attention
- Helps in building communication
- Builds interpersonal and intrapersonal relationship
- Balancing emotional well-being
- Develops coping strategies

The need of the hour is to enhance mindful listening and to respect everyone's emotions and feelings. Through this act, we can form meaningful relationships, and be better humans in general. The little act of recalling something someone told you is a spark of positivity we need in these dark times.

# 11

# THE HEALING POWER OF DANCING

"Consciousness expresses itself through creation. This world we live in is the dance of the creator. Dancers come and go in the twinkling of an eye but the dance lives on. On many occasion when I am dancing, I have felt touched by something sacred. In those moments, I felt my spirit soar and become one with everything that exists."

~ *Michael Jackson*

Dancing is more than just body movements and steps on the floor, it has amazing abilities to support physical and mental health. It is important to train and condition our body and dancing connects the body and soul, it is a door to all the positivities. Maratha Graham once said, "I feel that the essence of dance is the expression of man- the landscape of his soul. I hope that every dance I do reveals something of myself or some wonderful thing a human can be."

Dance promotes mental and physical wellness and holds a power of healing, it eliminates fatigue, stress, tensions, depression, etc. There is developing evidence that any form of dance promotes positive mental health. If we try and measure people's happiness before and after a dance performance, there would be an increase in the level of happiness after the dance. It is an integration with psychotherapy.

**Improves Mood and Reduces Anxiety-** Dance itself enhances the mood and eradicates worries and all the negative thoughts.

**Builds Physical and Mental Health-** Dance involves mind and body. It physically improves the body posture, eliminates pain, and aches, improves the immune system, solves body image issues, boosts metabolism, and builds resilient behaviour.

**Reflects Change-** There is a tendency to accept the change and move on by accepting things positively.

**Improves Cognitive Performance-** Certain parts of the brain get active and help in better thinking and improve memory.

Dance itself is a magic and vulnerable. The need of the hour is to embrace dancing and empower it and also understand that it promotes positive mental health.

Life is indeed challenging, but we need to learn to dance through it.

# 12

# GRIEF

"Grief is like the ocean; it comes in waves ebbing and flowing. Sometimes the water is calm and sometimes it is overwhelming. All we can do is learn to swim."

*~Vicki Harrison*

Grief is a response to loss; it is the experience that is faced mostly during the time of shock, trauma, and loss. Grief can disrupt psychological and physical well-being by making it difficult to think, connect with people, and cause change in sleeping and eating habits. Grieving differs on each individual; we all need to respect and support the process without passing any judgement or humiliating the individual because the healing happens only gradually.

Symptoms of grief:

- Denial- Unable to accept the situation and denying that there is a loss of someone or anything.
- Anger- Projecting anger on someone or oneself for no good reason and being resentful.

- Fear- Worries, anxiety, panic attacks, the trigger of fearing the loss of more people in the future.
- Guilt- Holding survivors guilt
- Sadness- Feelings of emptiness and loneliness may be a recurring hit

Other symptoms can be insomnia, profound weight loss or gain complains of aches and pains in the body, nausea, fatigue, dizziness, etc.

To ensure these symptoms do not get out of hand, always seek aid immediately. Also, if you know someone who is grieving, do keep an eye on them to ensure they do not take rash decision.

How to deal with grieving?

- We need to understand and acknowledge that grieving is normal, and healing happens only gradually. Accepting the fact that grieving can be a rush of different emotions is a start.
- Sharing with a loved one, seeking help from a therapist or counsellor, taking care of your own needs, paying keen attention to it spiralling to depression.

Grieving is normal, but when it spirals to the bottom side, feelings of worthlessness, suicidal tendencies, physically hurting oneself for the loss are common consequences, and all of these can be dangerous. It is always good to seek help from a therapist or a counsellor at this significant stage.

# 13

# RESILIENCE

"Out of suffering have emerged the strongest souls; the most massive characters are seared with scars."

~ *Khahil Gibran*

Resilience is one of the superpowers. Only with resilience can we deal with the chaos in life and to move smoothly personally as well as professionally. We need to stay rooted like the trees. How much ever storm it endures, we need to learn to surf through and stay rooted to the ground. We need to be optimistic in order to be resilient.

In life it is all about how we bounce back and cultivate resilience. All of us go through hardships and moments of sorrow and struggle. Resilience may be developed as a skill. We need to tackle each challenge as an opportunity to grow and mould our inner strength to cope with it. As Helen Killer said, "Although the world is full of suffering, it is also full of the overcoming it."

Resilience is what gives us the mental strength to thrive. Resilient people are better able to cope with the challenges in life in a better way, sort out any problems which may include financial trouble, divorce, relationship issues, death of a loved one, depression, trauma, etc. Those of them who lack resilience can go through an enormous amount of isolation when overwhelmed by the situation.

We can build resilience by reframing our negative thoughts into a positive one, seeking support, developing coping strategies, talking to those who are trustworthy, believing in yourself, by developing problem solving skills, embracing change, finding a purpose and to practicing other mindful ways of dealing with the hardships.

Focusing on practicing these skills can make a huge difference, it may be difficult in the beginning but as you adapt to it you will feel the magic in it, resilience acts as a magic wand, it's all in our hands how to make the best use of it.

# 14

# ART AS AN AID TO POSITIVE MENTAL HEALTH

"The aim of art is not to represent the outwards appearance of things, but their inward significance."

*~Aristotle*

Art possesses a magical healing power and helps in treating mental disorders and improves mental health. Art therapy is a form of expressive therapy which helps in dealing with many psychological disorders. Practicing art is like experimenting in a happiness laboratory. It helps in visually expressing oneself by contemplating the changes, triumphs, and trauma in one's life. It acts as a good painkiller.

The thoughts that have been lurking in the sub-conscious mind can be put across in the form of art. It is very important to know that to sketch, paint or to create any form of art we need not be expert or professional. Mental health professionals say that art comprises of many healing powers, like, reducing stress, boosting self-esteem, leading to self-discovery and also helps to fight stress, trauma, and depression. Creating art stimulates in the release of dopamine and releases the emotions that we have been holding inside.

Practicing art is easier if we will allow ourselves to explore its possibilities in promoting positive health. When creating art, you often channel your inner thoughts and emotions into the form and are left feeling fresh.

# 15

# IMPORTANCE OF CHILDREN'S MENTAL HEALTH DURING COVID-19

"A child's mental health is just as important as their physical health and deserves the same quality of support. No one would feel embarrassed about seeking help for a child if they broke their arm—and we really should be equally ready to support a child coping with emotional difficulties."

~ *Kate Middleton*

Everything in the world has been constantly changing since the spread of the COVID-19 pandemic. Lockdowns were declared in different parts of the world and has had drastic impact on our day to day lives, beginning from primary interactions in the family to the functioning of the global economy. It is important to prioritise the issue of mental health amidst the pandemic as more people are learning to adapt to take care of themselves and their loved ones during this stressful time.

The restrictions laid down due to the Covid-19 situation has been challenging to most individuals, but perhaps it is the children who have been affected the most. They have been quarantined within the four walls of their homes at a tender age when they should otherwise be playing and exploring outdoors with their friends like free birds. Due to this, children may experience feelings of uneasiness, confusion, anxiety, fear, loneliness, and stress. There may be changes in their behaviour as they become restless and bored with the monotonous routine. With schools being shut as a preventive measure, they remain isolated in their homes and away from their social circle. Studies have also shown an increase in screen time and reduced physical activity.

Different age groups face different issues. For example, Primary and secondary school kids may be detached from playing in the colony with friends or in school, adolescents may struggle to stay connected with their friends through social media, it may be difficult to explain to the pre-adolescent children why they cannot step outdoors to play anymore, new-born babies may experience a different set of issues as their upbringing will be limited to the individuals in the house and without the larger extended family and friends. Teenagers with phones may get addicted to it, college-going students may face anxiety with exams, entrance and other exams, and other relationship issues may also play an adverse role in their mental health.

The psychosocial support to children:

- **Parenting should be more open:** Parents should talk to the children freely and let the children talk to the parent freely, it is very important to pay attention to their behaviour and listen to them. Parents should choose their words wisely.
- **Keep them connected with their friends**: It's essential to keep the friend's circle connected so that they can have someone to share and have some fun time with each other.
- **Encourage them to take up new hobbies:** Parents should encourage them to try out and innovate new things. It helps them in exploring and embracing their creativity.

- **Get them a pet:** A pet at home always creates a positive atmosphere and also helps the child to be more empathetic towards others.
- **Teach them the do's and don'ts:** As a part of the important lesson in a child's life, teach them the rights and wrongs in life. The lessons parents teach their children are the steppingstones of life.
- **Monitor their internet usage:** To keep a track of internet use and also to keep a check on their use of social media is also the need of the hour.

Children's mental health is just as important as their physical health. Help them build resilience which will in turn help them to cope up with any problems. Parents or the caregiver should always encourage children to speak up and share, they should be reassured that the parent is always there to support and help them at any circumstance.

# 16

# NOMOPHOBIA: THE MODERN LIFE PHOBIA

"It has become appallingly obvious that our technology has exceeded our humanity."

~ *Albert Einstein*

Life today is the hub of the technological world, a day without it is hard to digest. Every one of us requires technology to survive in today's world. We are so much reliant on the phone that we use reminders to notify events, set alarms, store information etc.

Nomophobia (no-mobile-phone-phobia) is the feeling of distress or anxiety experienced in the absence of mobile phone. Addiction towards the mobile phone is rampant among all the age groups, even toddlers today require a mobile phone to keep themselves entertained or distract them while having meals. They tend to display adamant behaviour when restricted access to their tablets and phones. Nomophobia is 'new modern phobia', and it drastically impacts an individual;

1. Psychosocially: Loss of physical connection, loneliness, bereavement, social disruption, etc.
2. Physical Health: Headaches and migraines, itching eyes, heart diseases, skin allergies, etc.
3. Mental Health: Irritation, worry, depression, anxiety, etc.

Basically, it can be categorised as a serious disorder.

Symptoms of Nomophobia:

- Fear of turning off the phone
- Becoming anxious when there is low battery
- Constantly checking messages, calls, and emails or scrolling through social media frequently.
- Carrying the phone wherever they go
- Frequent checks if the phone is in hand or misplaced.

How to cope with this issue?

- Finding new and unique ways to occupy oneself: Trying creative ways and engaging with nature can help in keeping oneself engaged in a healthy activity.
- Set a time limit: There should be a limit to screen time, new apps can help in tracking the usage on each source in the mobile, also there are apps which freeze after a certain time and disables the use for a prolonged period.
- Take breaks- It's very important to take short breaks from your mobile so that there is also less stress to the eyes and also to overcome other problems.
- Engage yourself physically than virtually- To be connected physically creates a strong social bond and understanding between a peer group or individuals.

- By setting timers and looking away from the screen you can make a difference to yourself and the people around you. You can connect with people more as well as yourself.
- Taking a break from the phone and engaging in different activities does a lot of good for physical as well as emotional well-being. So, keep a check on your screen time and have control over its usage.

# 17

# DIFFERENCES BETWEEN DEPRESSION AND SADNESS

"Depression isn't just being a bit sad. It's feeling nothing. It's wanting to be not alive anymore."

~ *J.K Rowling*

In today's society, depression and sadness are both misunderstood. It's very important to know the difference between the two. Sadness hits every day of our life, but it all depends on the duration and intensity of the feelings, and it is seen in all the age groups. Depression and sadness are two faces of the same coin Prolonged sadness, say for more than 2 weeks, it can be termed as depression.

The actual difference between sadness and depression:

Sadness: It is the normal 'sad' or 'unhappy' feeling that is common in our daily routine. Sadness is when experiencing a low mood, and it lasts for less than 2 weeks. Some of them seek relief by crying it out or talking to someone about their problems on what is making them feel sad. Sadness is a process that slows down as time passes by.

Depression: It is a mental illness where the symptoms differ from sadness, like Insomnia, hopelessness, recurrent suicidal thoughts, irritability and fatigue, lack of motivation and self-harm. Depression can occur in a state of melancholy too (no identifiable cause). It is very important to pay a visit to a professional for help at this time, if not it may lead to a dire crisis of life.

How to support someone with the symptoms of depression?

- It's important to be sensitive
- Being non-judgemental
- Be empathetic
- Encourage them to speak up
- Mindful listening
- Observe the signs, especially if the individual is showing any suicidal tendencies.
- Know the treatment (therapy/counselling) options.

Some techniques to cope with depression:

- Connect socially- Forming a social network and engaging in healthy communication, sharing, and discussing with friends and family members can be helpful.
- Do something you like- Listening to music, gardening, cooking, reading books, taking care of a pet, these can help in distracting oneself from depressive thoughts.
- Get some sunlight- Getting out in nature and getting some sunlight sometime during the day is healthy and can improve the mood.
- Engage in household chores- Cleaning and making the house tidy, this involves moving which helps in some change in the mood though it is difficult to do so.

- Practice mindfulness- Being present at the moment is very important and being mindful of your surroundings helps in forgetting about the past and focus on today.

Do keep an eye on our for people you think are vulnerable or showing signs of depression. If you feel low, report to a close friend, family member or trusted individual.

With a professional help, there are different forms of medications and therapies like Psychotherapy, CBT (Cognitive behavioural therapy), DBT (Dialectical behavioural therapy), and many more that can help you tackle your depression.

Depression is a tax on human life, it can be life threatening. It is important to pay keen attention to our own feelings, mental health should be given the same amount of concern and respect as one gives to their physical health. It is important to seek professional help before it takes a toll on your life. As per a saying by Benjamin Franklin, "An ounce of prevention is worth a pound of cure."

# 18

# CONTROL YOUR ANGER, BEFORE IT CONTROLS YOU

"Holding on to anger is like grasping a hot coal with the intent of throwing it at someone else; you are the one who gets burned."

~ *Gautham Buddha*

We have all experienced anger, and it is absolutely normal to feel annoyed or angry. But it's destructive power can be catastrophic. Anger can be both external and internal, and there can be aggressive behaviour and passive-aggressive behaviour.

**Aggressive Behaviour-** Throwing temper tantrums verbally and non-verbally, resulting in a strong form of communication.

**Passive-Aggressiveness-** An anger expressed indirectly by being sarcastic hostile, criticizing, ignoring, or intentionally passing negative commentary.

Anger is one of the strongest emotions, how we react when angry not only impacts the individual himself/herself but also the surroundings. Hence it is very important to think before reacting, because it is said that when angry, we do not think about or words and actions expressed, and this can lead to more of suffering and feelings of guilt in the future. Those who get angry quickly tend to have a very low tolerance level, therefore it is important to control their anger.

Anger Management techniques:

- Learn to forgive – It is important to forgive and move on in life. Also, we need to understand that everyone is human. But when the individual regrets his or her mistake then we need to learn to forgive.
- Listen to music- Listening to music calms down and promotes a positive attitude.
- Take a break- Take a break when it's overwhelming and take a deep breath and relax.
- Write a gratitude journal- Practicing writing a gratitude journal helps in building positive energy.
- Laugh out- By forgetting all the negatives, we need to embrace all the positives.

To keep our anger in check and think before reacting is an important step. Try counting digits if you feel on the edge and watch how quickly you realise how harmful your future actions could have been.

# 19

# Problematic Gender Role Stereotyping

"You become a man by knowing victory and defeat, by running and crying. It's ok to cry...!! You can overcome."

~ *Euchiro Oda*

When was the last time you cried? Have you ever come cross a man crying, if yes what were your first thoughts about him? Is it ok for men to cry or is it associated with weakness?

Crying is a natural expression which all the living things on this earth experience. When in sadness, pain, grief or joy we tend to shed tears. Both men and women express emotions of crying, but in society crying is associated with gender roles. It is correlated to women and is seen as a weakness.

Gender roles play a very crucial role in shaping a human character, men are meant to suppress their feelings because of the social pressure, if men cry they are reprimanded and made fun of. "Don't cry like a girl" , "You're a man, you are supposed to be strong". Women are labelled as weak because they cry, a false assumption created by the society.

Children growing into adults carry the same mindset of thinking that 'Men are not meant to cry, only girls are said to be weak, so they cry', and men continue to suppress their emotions and suffer, unable to express.

So, it is important to understand that men also have an equal right to vent out their feelings which just as women do. We need to break the stereotyped thought that crying is weak and is only associated with the female gender.

Crying is also a stress buster. When shedding tears, you often expel the toxic feelings and find a medium to express your struggles. So, the next time you feel overwhelmed, let it out. Do not let anyone decide if you can cry or not.

# 20

# HOPE

"Hope is the thing with feathers that perches in the soul And sings the tune without the words and never stops at all."

~ *Emily Dickinson*

Hope means different things to different individuals. It is believed that hope is a positive assumption we have at different points in life but is hope really only about optimism or motivation that drives us? However, research in abundance has taught us how healthy hope can be and how important it is. From a youngster to an adult, the way we perceive hope changes. It's easier as a child and harder as an adult. As a child, hope drives stronger willpower and stronger motivation with shorter goals, on the other hand, as an adult our goals differ, our motivation gets shorter with a balance of responsibility and willpower trying to reach an ideal level.

How does one find hope in life? Hope is a path we choose to believe in. With hope comes responsibility, vision, and strength. Hope never comes as a gift to anyone but can surprise you in ways you didn't fathom. An article that I read on hope once said, "What happens to us at different stages of life is inevitable. What we can control is how we view them and accept them." Hope lies in the smallest action, the acceptance, to fight, to dream, to achieve, to plan.

Hope is as simple as waking up every morning believing that your time will come soon. It is what keeps the human mind and soul going even in the dreariest of times.

Hope does not limit to just the endpoints of our life or when defeating a bad situation, but it also helps in improving the quality of our life. Hope brings more mature outcome of understanding, openness, and acceptance. Hope being so subjective is something we all look forward to everyday consciously or unconsciously. Many have survived the pandemic caused by the Covid-19 in 2020 by living on hope and for the rest, hope became a wish.

It's believed, "Hope is a match in a dark tunnel, a moment of light, just enough to reveal the path ahead and ultimately the way out. "

So, never stop hoping. Keep your heart and always believe that something good will happen and soon enough it will.

# Meet The Authors

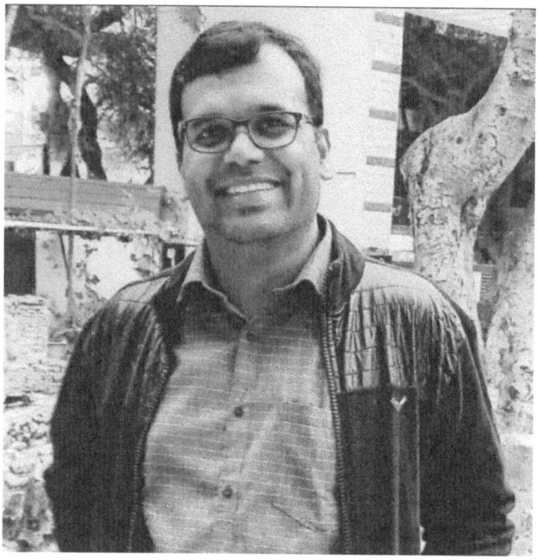

# PAUL RAJ

**Paul Raj** is an Assistant Professor of Psychology in Jyoti Nivas College Autonomous, Bengaluru. He has obtained a postgraduate degree in Counselling Psychology and M.Phil. in Learning Disabilities. Presently he is pursuing a PhD in Cognitive Functioning and Mathematical Abilities among Primary School Children and teaches courses in Basic Psychological Processes, Lifespan Development, Cognitive Psychology, and Positive Psychology, apart from guest lectures in Counselling Skills and Learning Disabilities. His research areas include child and adolescent development, specific learning disorders and positive psychology. He is also a practising Positive Psychotherapist in the areas related to children and adolescents.

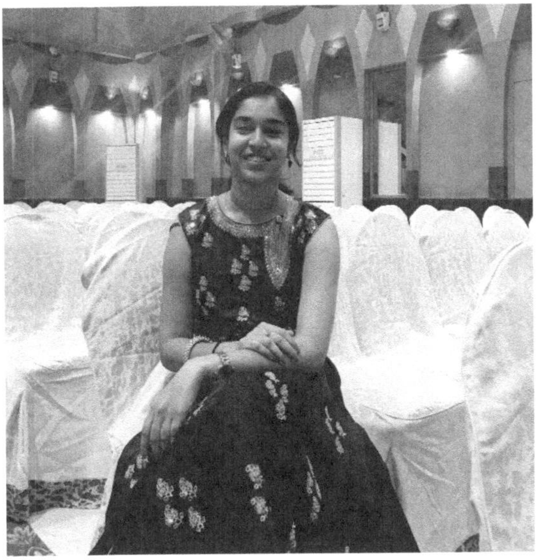

# AISHWARYA SIBEY

**Aishwarya Sibey** is presently pursuing her Master's in Psychology (MSc) from the Indian Institute of Psychology and Research (IIPR), Bengaluru. She is an outgoing President of Rotaract Club, Jyoti Nivas College Autonomous for the academic year, 2019-20. A passionate pet lover, a youth writer who writes poems, articles, and blogs. She exhibits her research interests in the areas of neurodevelopmental disorders, animal therapy, clinical psychology, criminal psychology, and positive psychology.

# ABOUT MINDSOLASTA

MindSolasta
think. change. illuminate.

In today's game of life positive psychology is at its peak. Mindsolasta helps the reader pause and reflect on the presence of positive aspects in daily life. Gratitude, mindfulness, hope, and stress management are some of the useful skills you will incorporate by reading this book. So, what are you waiting for? Dive right in to learn more about the secrets to a happier life and for a cup of positivity in your everyday life.

**Connect with us**

Mindsolasta

Mindsolasta

mindsolasta@gmail.com

www.mindsolasta.com